GALLSTONES

QUICKLY DEAL WITH THE FACTORS THAT CAUSE GALLSTONES

DR. LOGAN MONTGOMERY

Contents

CHAPTER ONE

INTRODUCTION

Gallstones are hardened deposits of digestive fluid that may shape in your gallbladder. Your gallbladder is a small, pear-shaped organ on the right aspect of your stomach, actually below your liver. The gallbladder holds a digestive fluid called bile it certainly is launched into your small intestine.

Gallstones are hardened deposits of bile that could form to your gallbladder. Bile is a digestive fluid produced on your liver and stored to your gallbladder. While you consume, your gallbladder contracts and empties bile into your small gut (duodenum).

Gallstones variety in length from as small as a grain of sand to as huge as a golf ball. A few human beings increase just one gallstone, on the equal time as others expand many gallstones on the identical time.

Folks that revel in symptoms from their gallstones commonly require gallbladder elimination surgical procedure. Gallstones that do not reason any signs and symptoms and signs typically don't want remedy.

Gallstones are hardened collections of bile substances that enlarge in your gallbladder. They can be as small as a grain of sand or as massive as a ping pong ball. Maximum don't purpose any troubles, however they are able to motive troubles in the event that they get loose and adventure into your bile ducts. The circumstance of having gallstones is called cholelithiasis.

Gallstones form in your gallbladder, the small, pear-formed organ in which your body shops bile. They're pebble-like quantities of targeted bile substances. Bile fluid contains cholesterol, bilirubin, bile salts and lecithin. Gallstones are usually manufactured from ldl cholesterol or bilirubin that acquire at the bottom of your gallbladder till they harden into "stones."

Gallstones may be as small as a grain of sand or as large as a golfing ball. They develop regularly, as bile continues to clean over them and that they accumulate more materials. Simply, it's the smaller stones which can be more likely to motive problem. That's because smaller stones can journey, at the identical time as larger ones have a tendency to stay put. Gallstones that tour may also get stuck somewhere and create a blockage.

Gallstones are portions of strong fabric that form for your gallbladder, a small organ under your liver. If you have them, you may listen your scientific health practitioner say you've got were given cholelithiasis.

Your gallbladder shops and releases bile, a fluid made in your liver, to help in digestion. Bile moreover includes wastes like ldl cholesterol and bilirubin, which your body makes at the same time as it breaks down purple blood cells. These things can form gallstones.

Gallstones can range in size from a grain of sand to a golf ball. You could not understand which you have them until they block a bile duct, causing pain that desires remedy right away.

Gallstones (biliary calculi) are small stones made from ldl cholesterol, bile pigment and calcium salts, normally in a combination that office work within the gallbladder. They may be a not unusual disease of the digestive device, and have an effect on round 15% of human beings elderly 50 years and over.

A few things which can reason gallstones to form consist of the crystallisation of more ldl cholesterol in bile and the failure of the gallbladder to empty surely.

In maximum times, gallstones don't motive any problems. However, you could want set off remedy if stones block ducts and purpose complications which includes infections or contamination of the pancreas (pancreatitis).

Surgeons may also additionally get rid of your gallbladder (known as a cholecystectomy) if gallstones (or extraordinary sorts of gallbladder ailment) are causing issues. Strategies embody laparoscopic ('keyhole') cholecystectomy or open surgical procedure. The gallbladder isn't a vital organ, so your frame can cope pretty nicely without it.

Gallstones may also motive no signs and signs or signs and symptoms. If a gallstone hotels in a duct and causes a blockage, the resulting symptoms and symptoms and signs and symptoms may embody:

Surprising and unexpectedly intensifying pain in the better proper a part of your abdomen

Unexpected and hastily intensifying ache inside the middle of your stomach, just below your breastbone

Returned ache amongst your shoulder blades

Ache for your proper shoulder

Nausea or vomiting

Gallstone ache may additionally final several minutes to three hours.

What's cholelithiasis?

Cholelithiasis is the situation of getting gallstones. Many humans have cholelithiasis and don't realise it. Gallstones received't always cause any issues for you. If they don't, you could leave them by myself. But gallstones can on occasion cause issues through developing a blockage. This will cause pain and contamination for your organs. If it's miles going untreated, it could purpose intense complications.

Gallstone types

The 2 essential forms of gallstones are:

Ldl cholesterol stones. These are commonly yellow-green. They are the maximum common, making up eighty% of gallstones.

Pigment stones. These are smaller and darker. They are made from bilirubin.

Reasons and chance factors for gallstones

Gallstones are extra commonplace in ladies than in men. They're moreover extra not unusual in folks that are overweight and those with a own family statistics of gallstones.

There can be no single cause of gallstones.

In a few humans, the liver produces too much ldl cholesterol. This can bring about the formation of ldl cholesterol crystals in bile that develop into stones. In other humans, gallstones shape because of changes in different components of bile or because the gallbladder does no longer empty generally.

Make an appointment along with your health practitioner when you have any symptoms or symptoms that fear you.

Are searching for on the spot care in case you boom signs and symptoms and signs and signs of a excessive gallstone problem, along with:

Belly pain so severe which you can't take a seat though or find a secure characteristic

Yellowing of your pores and skin and the whites of your eyes (jaundice)

Excessive fever with chills

How does having gallstones (cholelithiasis) have an impact on me?

Your gallbladder is part of your biliary device. It belongs to a community of organs that pass bile amongst every distinct. Those organs are associated via a chain of pipelines known as bile ducts. Bile travels via the bile ducts from your liver on your gallbladder, and out of your gallbladder in your small intestine. Your pancreas also makes use of the bile ducts to deliver its personal digestive juices.

A gallstone that travels to the mouth of your gallbladder can hinder the drift of bile in or out. A gallstone that makes its manner from your gallbladder and into the bile ducts should block the go with the flow of bile via the ducts. This may cause bile to lower again up into the close by organs. Even as bile backs up, it builds strain and pain for your organs and bile ducts and reasons contamination.

This could lead to a spread of complications, such as:

Gallbladder ailment. Gallstones are the maximum commonplace reason of gallbladder illnesses. Once they get caught, they motive bile to back up into your gallbladder, causing contamination. This could do long-term harm for your gallbladder over the years, scarring the tissues and preventing it from functioning. The stalled go together with the waft of bile additionally makes infections on your gallbladder much more likely.

Liver illness. A blockage everywhere within the biliary machine can reason bile to again up into your liver. This will purpose irritation to your liver, leading to an extended chance of infection and lengthy-time period scarring over the years (cirrhosis). If your liver stops functioning properly, your entire biliary device breaks down. You could stay without a gallbladder but now not with out a liver.

Gallstone pancreatitis. A gallstone that

blocks the pancreatic duct will cause inflammation in your pancreas. As along side your exclusive organs, temporary infection causes ache, and chronic infection reasons lengthy-time period harm that can stop your organ from functioning.

Cholangitis. Contamination on your bile ducts can cause infections within the quick time period and scarring within the long time. Scarring in your bile ducts causes them to narrow, which restricts the flow of bile. This could motive lengthy-term bile-go along with the glide issues even after the blockage has been removed.

Jaundice. Subsidized-up bile will leak into your bloodstream, making you ill. Bile includes pollution that your liver has filtered from your frame. The bilirubin content has a yellow color, as a way to be seen inside the whites of your eyes.

Malabsorption. If bile can't journey to your small gut as supposed, you may have problem breaking down and absorbing nutrients from your food. Bile is specially critical for breaking down fat and for soaking up fat-soluble nutrients for your small gut.

Gallstone hazard elements

You're much more likely to get gallstones if you:

Have a family records of them

Are a girl

Are over age 40

Are of native American or Mexican descent

Are obese

Have a food regimen excessive in fat and ldl ldl cholesterol however low in fiber

Don't get masses exercising

Use starting manage capsules or hormone replacement therapy

Are pregnant

Have diabetes

Have an intestinal sickness like Crohn's

Have hemolytic anemia or cirrhosis of the liver

Take medicinal drug to decrease your ldl ldl cholesterol

CHAPTER TWO

Lose masses of weight in a short time

Are fasting

Diagnosis of gallstones

Scientific docs diagnose gallstones through the usage of some of checks, consisting of:

Fashionable checks – which includes physical examination and x-rays

Ultrasound – soundwaves shape a image that indicates the presence of gallstones

Endoscope check – endoscopic retrograde cholangiopancreatography (ERCP). A skinny tube is surpassed through the oesophagus and injects dye into the bowel to enhance the satisfactory of x-ray pictures

Hepatobiliary iminodiacetic acid (HIDA) test – a unique form of nuclear test that assesses how properly the gallbladder features

Magnetic resonance cholangiopancreatography (MRCP) – a form of the body-imaging approach magnetic resonance imaging (MRI). The liver, biliary and pancreatic machine is imaged the use of an MRI unit. The image is much like an ERCP take a look at.

Complications of gallstones

If gallstones reason no symptoms, you no longer regularly want any treatment.

Complications which can require prompt medical remedy embody:

Biliary colic – a gallstone can circulate from the body of the gallbladder into its neck (cystic duct), primary to obstruction. Signs consist of excessive pain and fever

Contamination of the gallbladder (cholecystitis) – a gallstone blocks the gallbladder duct, principal to infection and contamination of the gallbladder. Signs and symptoms and symptoms include intense belly pain, nausea and vomiting

Jaundice – if a gallstone blocks a bile duct main to the bowel, trapped bile enters the person's bloodstream in place of the digestive machine. The bile pigments reason a yellowing of the man or woman's skin and eyes. Their urine may moreover flip orange or brown

Pancreatitis – inflammation of the pancreas, due to a blocked bile duct low down near the pancreas. Pancreatic enzymes aggravate and burn the pancreas and leak out into the stomach cavity

Cholangitis – infection of the bile ducts, which occurs even as a bile duct will become blocked through a gallstone and the bile will become infected. This reasons pain, fever, jaundice and rigors (shaking)

Infection of the liver

Most cancers of the gallbladder (takes place now not regularly).

Does cholelithiasis require surgical operation?

The majority with gallstones will by no means need treatment. But if your gallstones motive troubles, your healthcare company will want to get rid of them. Commonly, they'll want to do away with all your gallstones, even supposing most effective taken into consideration considered one of them is currently causing problem. If a blockage happens as soon as, it's in all likelihood to arise once more. The threat isn't truly really worth ready around for.

Because of the reality there's no way to get right of entry to the gallstones internal your gallbladder without disposing of it, the same old treatment for complicated gallstones is to cast off the gallbladder absolutely. That may be a minor surgical treatment, and you may live well with out a gallbladder. If you have gallstones on your bile ducts, your healthcare business enterprise will ought to remove the ones one by one as properly.

Can gallstones leave without surgical treatment?

Gallstones for your bile ducts that aren't caught can efficiently bypass via them and into your intestines. You can skip them out via your poop. It's far a lucky state of affairs, but in popular, you don't need to chance having gallstones for your bile ducts in the first location. In the occasion that they don't bypass all of the manner out of you, they will simplest grow large over the years.

There are a few medicinal tablets that might assist to dissolve smaller gallstones. The ones take many months to artwork, so that they aren't the most practical alternative for humans experiencing symptoms. But they provide an opportunity for people who may not be in a relaxed fitness situation for surgical procedure. They will also be realistic for human beings who have gallstones but don't have signs but.

How are gallstones eliminated?

There are a few specific techniques to put off gallstones.

Endoscopy

Gallstones on your bile ducts are eliminated thru endoscopy (ERCP). This doesn't require any incisions. The gallstones pop out through the prolonged tube that's been exceeded down your throat. Gallstones to your gallbladder are removed via using casting off the gallbladder (cholecystectomy). This will typically be carried out through laparoscopy, a minimally-invasive surgical treatment approach.

Laparoscopy

A laparoscopic cholecystectomy makes use of small, "keyhole incisions" to your stomach to feature with the resource of a small digital camera called a laparoscope. Your health care expert inserts the laparoscope through one keyhole and gets rid of your gallbladder via another. Smaller incisions make for less put up-operative pain and a quicker recovery time than traditional, "open" surgical remedy.

Open surgical treatment

A few human beings may additionally additionally have more complex conditions that require open surgical treatment to govern. If you have open surgical treatment, you'll have an extended health center stay in some time and an prolonged recuperation at home to your large incision. Some laparoscopic cholecystectomies also can want to convert to open surgical operation in case your healthcare expert runs into headaches at some stage in the way.

Prevention

You could reduce your hazard of gallstones in case you:

Do no longer skip food. Try to keep on with your normal mealtimes every day. Skipping meals or fasting can boom the risk of gallstones.

Shed pounds slowly. If you need to shed pounds, go slow. Rapid weight loss can growth the danger of gallstones. Purpose to lose 1 or 2 pounds (approximately 0.Five to at least one kilogram) a week.

Eat greater excessive-fiber ingredients. Embody greater fiber-rich meals for your weight loss program, including culmination, vegetables and whole grains.

Preserve a wholesome weight. Weight problems and being overweight boom the risk of gallstones. Paintings to benefit a wholesome weight by way of way of reducing the wide kind of strength you consume and increasing the quantity of physical interest you get. After you advantage a healthful weight, work to hold that weight through continuing your healthy weight loss program and persevering with to workout.

CONCLUSION

Gallstones are commonplace, and most of the people will in no manner be bothered with the resource of them. If they live hooked up your gallbladder, you'll probably in no way realise they're there. But after they start to skip, they come to be volatile. Those tiny, pebble-like portions can do an entire lot of harm once they get into the tight areas of your sensitive biliary tool.

A gallbladder attack can be intense and frightening, specially if you didn't recognise you had gallstones initially. It can be alarming to find out that the advocated treatment is surgery. However laparoscopic gallbladder elimination is a commonplace technique with an first-rate diagnosis. Your entire ordeal may be over inside hours of your first signs and symptoms.

THE END

www.ingramcontent.com/pod-product-compliance
Lightning Source LLC
Chambersburg PA
CBHW060824260726
48660CB00003B/1082